How to Live Healthy and Stay Fit Even At 50

Advanced Health and Wellness Habits for Men and Women, Arthritis Pain Relief, Acne Treatment Secrets, Natural Remedies for Depression

Ronald Luke N.

Copyright

Table of contents

Introduction

I remember that day vividly. I stood in front of the mirror, disgusted by what I saw looking back at me. The man peering through bloodshot eyes, with a soft chin and swollen belly, was someone I didn't even recognize anymore.

I used to be active, fit and full of life. What really happened? How did I look this bad?

Now I was exhausted after a casual walk up the stairs and winded tying my own shoes. I avoided photos and weighed myself as little as possible because I didn't want to face the depressing truth of what I'd become.

Deep down, I knew this wasn't a physical problem - it was a mental and emotional crisis. Years of neglecting my health through poor diet, lack of movement and toxic stress had taken their toll. But I'd tried fix after fix - diets, supplements, gym memberships - desperate for a magic pill to solve my problems without real effort or sacrifice. No wonder nothing stuck.

That day, staring into the eyes of a stranger, I vowed this had to change. I was only 35 but felt a decade older. If I didn't take control right now, who knew how much worse it could get or if it would be too late?

I promised myself never to give up again. I was going to find an approach that didn't feel like constant suffering or sacrifice. One I could sustain for life, not just for a few months.

Luckily, I discovered a lifestyle method grounded in science that finally gave me sustainable results and a newfound sense of health and vitality. And that transformation changed my life in ways I never imagined.

If you're ready for a change like I was, keep reading to discover how to reclaim your health, energy and confidence from the inside out. It's time to address these health challenges and take total control of your well-being.

Description

Discover the Hidden Secrets to Transform Your Health and Lose Weight for Good. Are you tired of trying diet after diet only to gain the weight back plus more?

Frustrated with lack of lasting results from the fitness programs and workouts you've tried? You're not alone - millions struggle every day with their health goals.

But what if I tell you there was a simple, proven and effective way to finally take control of your health that didn't require deprivation or extreme workouts?

In this groundbreaking book, leading health expert John Doe shares the lifestyle secrets that have helped thousands permanently lose weight and transform their health.

In this book, you'll discover:

- The #1 myth about diets and weight loss that's holding most people back from success.

- The surprising connection between your daily habits and long-term health that no one talks about.

- A 5-minute daily "startup" ritual that helps melt pounds without adding more exercise.

- How to reprogram your thought patterns to stay motivated for the long haul.

- Strategies for dealing with cravings, temptations and plateaus so you keep moving towards your goals.

Packed with successful stories, and simple exercises, this book provides an easy-to-follow roadmap to better health that works.

Say goodbye to strict dieting and hello to the body and life you've always desired.

This book will transform your life for good. Don't delay! Get your copy...

Chapter 1

Getting Started with a Healthy Lifestyle

Changing a few simple things about your life can make you healthier, happier, and more successful. You will have to change everything about yourself, not just how much you work out or what you eat. The key to being happy and healthy is to keep your body and mind in balance.

We are only truly healthy when our physical, mental, and spiritual health are all in balance. If we're healthy, we're happier and more likely to be successful. Here are some ways to bring harmony and balance back into your life.

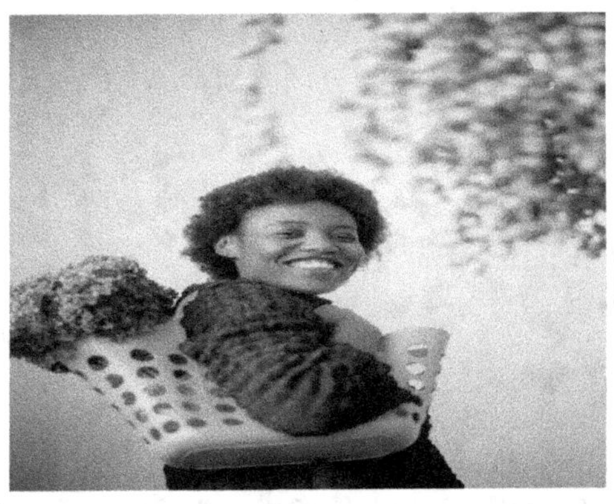

Exercise is important because it tones our muscles, keeps our hearts and lungs healthy, and rids our bodies of toxins. Exercise can be anything from more intense activities like aerobics to something as simple as walking.

Choose your favorite activity and set aside a certain time each day to work on getting your body back in shape. The next most important thing to do for a balanced life is to eat well. Our bodies need the right amount of vitamins, nutrients, and minerals to work at their best.

A Happier, More Successful, and Healthier you

It's easy to make changes to our diet. Just stay away from fast food, which is high in saturated fats and sugar, and eat more whole grains, chicken, fish, and lots of green vegetables.

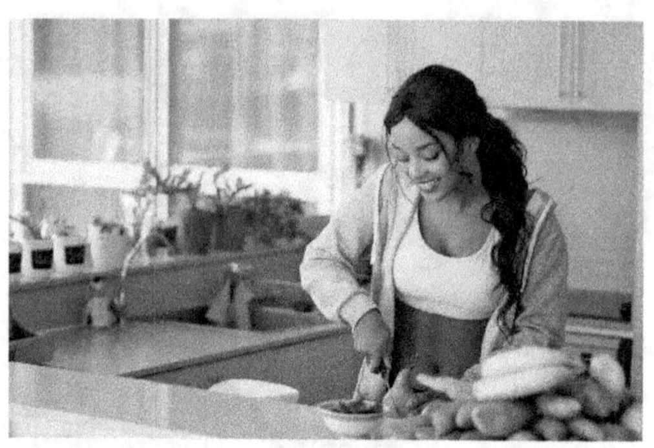

When fresh fruit is available, try to eat that instead of juice. Along with making changes to your diet, you should take vitamins, minerals, and other supplements. Many of the foods we eat now don't have the minerals our bodies need because of how they are grown. Instead, they only give us the basic nutrients we need.

Because of this, we might not be getting enough of some minerals and vitamins. We can make sure we still get all the important minerals, nutrients, and vitamins we need by taking vitamin and mineral supplements.

Reducing the amount of stress in our lives is a big part of how well we can deal with it. Stress can hurt our bodies and minds in many ways. It has been linked to burnout, tiredness, trouble sleeping, depression, and a weaker immune system.

Learning how to deal with stress and worry is important if you want to stay healthy and full of energy. There are many techniques, from simple breathing exercises that can be done anywhere and at any time to yoga, which is a full system for relaxing and getting rid of stress, to meditation. There are many books, DVDs, and CDs on the subject, and you can also take a course.

Last, but not least, it's important to keep life fun and do something every day that you enjoy and that makes you feel calm and happy. No, you are not being selfish when you take time for yourself every day. This time is important.

It's just as important as working out, eating well, and reducing stress. You could spend your time doing something you enjoy, like sitting quietly and reading, taking a hot bubble bath while listening to your favorite music, or spending quality time with your family or friends. It could be anything, as long as it's something you enjoy doing.

13 Ways to Get Healthier

1. The most important thing you can do to improve your health is to admit that you need to make adjustments to get healthier and more fit. Here are some tips to help you get healthier and become a better version of yourself.

2 Make it a goal to have a healthier outlook on life, which will make you healthier. If you are

determined to get healthier, it will be a lot easier to do so.

3. Back up your new way of thinking by learning as much as you can about ways to get healthier and live a healthier life. You can learn about healthy living from the internet, books, DVDs, clubs, gyms, and support groups. Knowing as much as you can about healthy living gives you a great place to start.

4. You have to start somewhere, so look at your kitchen and clean it up to get ready for your new way of life. Rearrange your kitchen cabinets, cupboards, and fridge so there are no reminders of the old you and only things that will help you in your new life.

5. Replace your old food with your new, healthier food, and don't forget to buy any small appliances, like blenders and food scales, that you will need to help you eat healthier.

6. Get a big planner calendar, hang it in your kitchen, and mark the day you decide to start your new lifestyle. Then, no matter what happens, you'll stick to it.

7. Keep a journal from the start. You can do this by hand or on your computer. You should write down everything you think and feel about your new ways and everything you notice has changed about yourself.

This is important to look back on so you can see how things are getting better because of your positive attitude and the changes you have made.

8). Positive thoughts, self-talk, or affirmations are a must; they will give you confidence at first and help you get through the hard times that will happen during the early changes.

9). In addition to making changes to your diet, you will also have to make changes to the amount of exercise you do every day. While good, healthy food is important, exercise is just as important because it can help prevent diseases like heart disease and help us lose weight or tone up.

10). Give up bad habits like smoking or drinking. You'll never be at your healthiest best as long as you're puffing on cigarettes or drinking regularly.

11) Make sure you eat the recommended five servings of fruit and vegetables every day. Fruit and vegetables are full of vitamins that your body needs.

12). Make sure you learn how to get rid of as much stress as you can from your life. There are many ways to do this, and one of them is sure to work for you.

13). If you cut out too much salt, sugar, and fat from your diet, your cholesterol and blood pressure will go down.

Important Notes about Food

The United States Department of Agriculture is the best place to start taking notes about nutrition (USDA). The USDA advises the general public about what they think are healthy eating habits.

And their information focuses on these main areas:
- Nutrition pyramid
- Needed nutrients
- Weight management
- Physical fitness and
- Food safety.

Nutrition Pyramid
The USDA has updated its dietary guidelines and added a food pyramid with a color scheme to help people eat healthily.

Needed Nutrients
In their nutrition pyramid, the USDA tells people to drink and eat a wide range of nutrient-dense drinks and foods from the main food groups. They also say to cut back on alcohol, salt, added sugars, cholesterol, saturated fats, and trans fats.

And they suggest following plans like the Dietary Approaches to Stop Hypertension (DASH) Eating Plan or the USDA Food Guide.

Weight Management

The USDA says that people should try to keep their weight in a healthy range by balancing the calories they get from food and drinks with the calories they burn. And as people get older, they should gradually cut back on the amount of food and drinks they eat and drink and get more physically fit.

Physical Fitness

The USDA wants people to be physically active regularly and do less sitting around. This is to promote not only healthy bodies but also overall health and mental well-being. Depending on your age, weight, and eating habits, the best amount of activity is between 30 and 90 minutes a day of moderate to intense physical activity.

Instead of just 30 minutes, most people should do a combination of more intense activity and/or longer periods of activity to get even more health benefits. Check with your doctor first to make sure this is okay.

Stretching exercises help you become more flexible. Cardiovascular conditioning and calisthenics or resistance exercises help you get stronger and have more endurance.

Food Safety

The USDA says that people can avoid getting sick from microorganisms in food by washing their hands, surfaces where they handle food, and vegetables and fruits well.

They also say not to wash meats and poultry, but you should keep raw foods separate from cooked or ready-to-eat foods when you shop, handle, and store food. They also say that foods should be cooked at temperatures high enough to kill microorganisms and that perishable foods should be put in the fridge or freezer right away.

Foods to Avoid

- Raw or uncooked milk
- Products made with milk that hasn't been pasteurized
- Raw or only half-cooked eggs
- Foods that have raw eggs in them
- Meat and poultry that is raw or not fully cooked
- Unpasteurized juices Sprouted seeds.

19

Chapter 2

How to Look Good and Feel Better

Feeling good on the inside can be a direct result of feeling good about ourselves, and vice versa. When we receive positive feedback about our appearance, it can improve our confidence and make us feel good about ourselves.

Dieting, eating a balanced diet, exercising, and generally taking care of one's physical and mental health are all effective methods for improving both outward appearance and internal well-being.

Stay Fit
Exercising regularly not only aids in weight loss but also tones your muscles, making you look and feel better and increasing your resistance to illness.

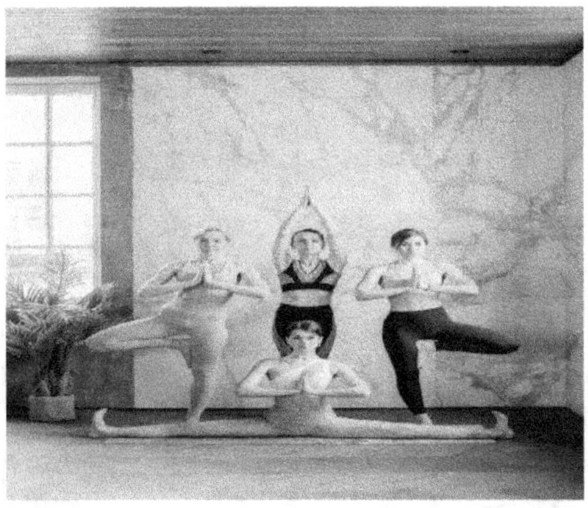

You can buy inexpensive basic gym equipment to use in the comfort of your own home, or you can take up a remarkable activity that costs you nothing at all: walking. If you want to stay in tip-top shape, a good diet, and regular exercise — ideally 30 minutes a day, seven days a week — are essential.

Healthy Eating

Eating fresh fruit and vegetables, which are full of vitamins and minerals, and eating at regular intervals is the foundation of a healthy, well-balanced diet.

Cutting back on meals high in salt, fat, and carbohydrates is important for keeping a healthy body and can help you lose weight if you are trying to eat fewer calories than you expend each day.

Bread, cereals, fish, lean meat, poultry, potatoes, and dairy products are all regarded staples of a healthy, well-balanced diet that, when combined with regular exercise, may do wonders for your appearance and health.

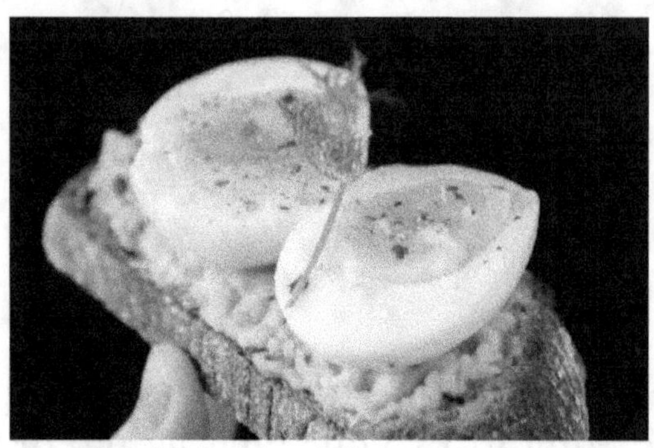

Several seemingly insignificant details contribute to how you look when you're taking care of your body as a whole. For instance, if you've been wearing the same hairdo for a while, getting a new cut and color can do wonders for your confidence.

Your hands and feet will thank you for visiting a manicurist or pedicurist, and your grin will thank you for having your teeth whitened.

When trying to improve your outward appearance, it's important to remember that it's the sum of many small changes that ultimately matters.

Take Care of Your Mental Health
The state of your mind, your emotions, and your thoughts can also have a significant impact on your overall well-being.

If you tend to dwell on the negative, your viewpoint will be negative as well, diminishing your confidence and damaging your sense of who you are.

Affirmations are a great way to increase your confidence and alter the way you think about yourself daily.

When taken together, these factors can help you become a healthier, happier person who is not only more physically fit and mentally resilient but also more attractive and self-confident on the outside.

Why It's Important to Maintain a Healthy Weight

Not only can extra weight make you look and feel unattractive, but it also puts your health at risk. For this and many other reasons, you must eat sensibly and engage in regular physical activity to keep your weight in the healthy range.

People who are overweight and don't exercise regularly have a higher risk of developing depression than those who do exercise regularly and eat a well-balanced, varied diet, suggesting that being overweight is associated with a wide range of conditions that can negatively impact both our physical and mental health.

It is widely accepted in the medical community that the more overweight a person is, the greater their risk of developing serious health problems; however, this risk decreases significantly after the person takes active efforts to begin losing weight and making adjustments to their lifestyle.

If you are overweight, you can begin to improve your health and lessen the dangers of it by dropping as little as 10 or 20 pounds. If any of the following apply to you and you are overweight, you should seriously consider losing weight.

Those who are genetically predisposed to certain chronic diseases, such as heart disease and diabetes, tend to be overweight themselves.

Are there Any Existing Health Problems?

Obesity-related illnesses include hypertension, high cholesterol, and diabetes. Being shaped like an apple, an increased risk of diabetes, various types of cancer, and heart disease is associated with carrying extra weight around the midsection.

- Weight-related diseases

Gallstones and other gallbladder issues Hypertensive Disorders the Risk of Getting Cancer Consequences of Diabetes The onset of gout Creating respiratory issues include sleep apnea, which causes breathing to stop repeatedly during sleep. Asthma, bronchitis, and other respiratory illnesses.

- Gallbladder Problem

Gallstones are a common concern in someone who is overweight and can cause serious issues for the obese. It is unclear why obesity has this effect on the gallbladder.

- Heart Disease

The leading cause of and a major risk factor in cardiovascular disease and stroke is high blood pressure, and being overweight increases your risk of developing hypertension by a factor of two.

Angina, which manifests as chest pain due to a lack of oxygen reaching the heart, is a disorder that can be exacerbated by obesity. Death from a stroke can occur suddenly and without warning if a person is extremely overweight or obese.

- Diabetes

Those who are overweight are twice as likely to develop type 2 diabetes as those who maintain a healthy weight, and being overweight is associated with an increased risk of death, cardiovascular disease, and vision loss.

- Reducing Your Cholesterol

Cholesterol levels should be monitored regularly, and a healthy range should be maintained, for optimal health. To keep cholesterol levels within the recommended range and ward against diseases like heart disease, we can make use of a wide variety of cholesterol-lowering strategies. These are some proven strategies for reducing cholesterol.

How Changes in Diet Can Help Reduce Cholesterol Levels

You should expend at least as many calories as you consume every day. Get at least 30 minutes of physical activity on most days of the week. Consume a wide range of nutrient-dense foods. Eat at least five servings of fruits and vegetables every day.

Increase your intake of high-fiber, whole-grain foods. At least twice weekly, seafood should be a part of your meal plan. Eliminate calorie- and nutrient-poor foods from your diet. Reduce your consumption of trans fats and saturated fats.

Take the skin off of the chicken and stick to lean cuts of meat. Limit your dairy intake to nonfat and low-fat varieties alone. Eliminating partly hydrogenated vegetable oil from your diet is an effective way to lower your intake of trans fats. Eat extremely little salt or none at all. Moderate alcohol consumption is recommended.

- Always check food labels for nutritional information:

Regular exercise can help you maintain healthy cholesterol levels; here are some suggestions for getting started.

Take it easy at first, but aim for 30 minutes of exercise per day. If at all feasible, try to incorporate your daily workout into your daily routine by performing it at the same time each day.

Be sure to stay hydrated by drinking plenty of water. Join a gym or train alongside a friend to make your exercise sessions more enjoyable. Document your exercise routine and the positive effects it has on your life.

Use the stairs instead of the elevator, park further away, and ride your bike or walk to the office. Switch up your exercise by doing something different every day. Stop exercising until you feel better; continue when you are healthy enough to do so.

If you want to maintain your cholesterol levels low, changing your lifestyle is essential; here are some things you can do:

See a doctor for guidance on your diet and exercise routine. If you want to know how much fat, sodium, and other substances are in the food you're buying, it's important to read the labels. If you are a smoker or alcoholic, please give up.

Why Weight Watchers are Ineffective

We've all heard of Weight Watchers, and those of us who've battled with diets to shed a few pounds might have additionally tried going to meetings. Some people have success there, while many others utterly fail.

There is no magic technique that will enable us to lose weight overnight while we sleep; instead, success with weight watchers depends entirely on the individual, just like with any other type of dieting.

Why do so many of us fail when it comes to dieting and adhering to a program like Weight Watchers? Knowing why any diet does not work is crucial for success, and the Weight Watchers program is no exception.

- Sticking to the plan

The largest error that most of us make is failing to keep to the plan. As Weight Watchers need a membership fee, you must have the dedication required to start the plan and see it through by sticking to it before enrolling.

The success of Weight Watchers depends on the individual maintaining track of their diet and utilizing all of the support that Weight Watchers offer to members. All diets essentially rely on keeping track of how many calories or point each food has, and Weight Watchers uses a points system where each food is given a value based on how many calories and fat grams it contains.

A person is then given a certain number of points throughout the day based on their weight and sex. The system will, of course, function effectively if the number of points is adhered to, but if the person consistently exceeds the suggested daily allotment of points, they will, quite simply, not lose weight and may even gain weight.

- Not keeping a journal

Keep a journal, list all the things you eat throughout the day, and keep track of all the points you consume for a program like Weight Watchers to be effective. Relying solely on your memory to keep track is not sufficient.

If you want to succeed with the Weight Watchers program, you must keep a written notebook in which you record every point you make, not just if you simply forget you ate something or whether you conveniently forget about the snack you had with your coffee.

- Guesswork

They overestimate the number of points they have consumed throughout the day, which is one of the main reasons why so many individuals struggle with Weight Watchers.

Guessing the number of points in a plateful of food puts you on the path to failure because you can never expect to lose weight if you consistently underestimate the number of points you are consuming.

The fact that some meals, including vegetables, have no points as long as you measure that amount in one cup causes some people who use the weight watcher's method to have misconceptions about the system.

Yet, they are taught to believe that you may eat as many veggies as you like and they would still count as zero points. As a result, some people believe that they are allowed to consume an endless quantity of these foods, which is false.

Always make sure you fully comprehend a program's points system, such as that of Weight Watchers, and if you have any questions, ask a representative for guidance on how to calculate using the points system.

Weight Watchers is no exception; to succeed in your weight loss program, you must have the willpower and drive required offorny diet.

Making the program work requires accurate point calculations, keeping a written record of everything you eat, sticking with it over time, and modifying your lifestyle and eating habits after you have successfully dropped the desired amount of weight.

Chapter 3

7 Effective Ways to Shed Ten Pounds in a Few Weeks

To look good for an approaching family function or another occasion, to feel better and fit into your clothes, or simply to look better, you may want to jumpstart a fitness routine or drop some weight.

It really would be good to shed 10 pounds quickly for them and any other occasions. Help is available in the shape of advice from experts who have already done it. So, get to work and drop 10!

- Create Time

Stop citing justifications! There is no better time to lose weight than right now because your health and fitness are priorities. You are not intending to achieve this if you don't set aside time and include exercise goals in your regular daily agenda.

Grab your day planner and calendar, then block off at least 30 minutes each day for exercising and engaging in physical activity.

- Create a Big Attack Plan

Secondly, do some research and make a plan of action for those excess fat pounds. You can pick from a variety of well-known fitness and weight loss programs, including Jenny Craig, Slim-Fast, the Mayo Clinic Plan, Atkins, Bill Phillips Body for Life, Weight Watchers, and more.

Alternatively, you can visit your neighborhood gym, engage a trainer, or simply start exercising on your own while keeping track of reps and resistance for better strength and endurance training.

- Mental Attitude

Change your mentality to have a constructive, wholesome perspective on your fitness objectives. Visit your local library to get motivating and inspirational books, audio cassettes, CDs, films, and articles to help you develop this mentality and maintain it throughout your program.

Also, search the Internet for useful resources including articles, ezines, audio and other file types, videos, eBooks, reports, and training.

- Change Your Diet

Establishing a healthy diet or selecting a healthy diet plan will help you take control of your nutritional demands. A nice site to search online is eDiets.com, which links up numerous well-known diet regimens for you and provides recipes.

A group chat room where people can connect online, plan meals, keep journals, and much more. For further resources, visit the library and other online dietary and nutritional sites.

- Follow Your Success Path

Take a notebook with you as you go towards your objectives and beyond. Write down your goals, the deadline, and the steps you plan to take to achieve them, such as exercising for 30 minutes each day and adhering to the Weight Watchers program's dietary restrictions.

- Exercise with Friends

Make friends and provide one another encouragement as you go. Get free chat rooms by searching for fitness forums on the Internet.

- Establish realistic objectives:

Be honest and concentrate on what functions finest, such as dropping 2 pounds weekly. When weight loss is accelerated, the pounds frequently end up coming back.

Helping Others with Your Weight Loss Plan

If you have developed and successfully followed a weight loss plan, you should share your strategy and achievement with others who are attempting to achieve your level of accomplishment.

Nothing helps people stick with a plan and accomplish it like motivation, and if they see it working, they are more likely to want to keep with a plan themselves and experience the same success in their lives.

The main reason weight loss groups like weight watchers have such a high success rate is that members share and encourage one another.

Just knowing that you are not the only person out there who is struggling and needs to lose weight may make a significant impact and build confidence.

If your weight-reduction plan has worked for you, what can you do to spread the word and encourage others to do the same? Here are some suggestions to get you going.

- Publish a blog

A lot of websites now offer free blog space, which is wonderful for disseminating your knowledge. The Internet is a great location to write a blog since it helps you to get your views and ideas out there to millions of people across the world.

A blog can be compared to an online journal; it's your place to express ideas, feelings, and thoughts, and you can share it with the entire globe by word of mouth. Share your effective weight reduction strategy on your blog and include a detailed account of all the steps you did to get to where you are now.

To persuade them that dieting can be successful, you can mention the plan you utilized, your exercise regimens, the menus you followed, as well as your sentiments and ideas.

- Organize regular meetings

If you have a group of friends who want to start a diet, get together and rent a community center once a week, or alternate hosting meetings in various homes each week.

When you meet together once a week, you can all weigh in at the same time, discuss your week's highlights, and encourage those who struggled.

Maintain written records for each group member and chart your progress each week. If one of you has had exceptional success in the past with your weight loss plan, you might be the one to take the lead and motivate the other participants to follow your example.

- Publish an ebook

Consider publishing a little ebook about your experiences and achievements if your weight loss strategy has been extremely successful to inspire others.

All computers have word processing software, so it doesn't need to be anything fancy. Start by organizing from the introduction, then read through the various chapters, and when you're done, print it off and give it to your friends.

It's a fantastic, enjoyable way to share your success story and offer them whatever encouragement they might require.

Chapter 4

How to Get Healthy by Mere Walking

The finest workout you can do to improve your health and physical fitness is walking, which costs you nothing. Everyone can engage in it, regardless of age or physical condition, as long as they start cautiously, just like with any sort of exercise they are not accustomed to.

If you don't exercise frequently, it's best to start with no more than a 10-minute walk most days of the week as your first step towards becoming healthier. Afterward, this can be gradually raised to walking twice daily for 15 minutes or three times daily for 10 minutes.

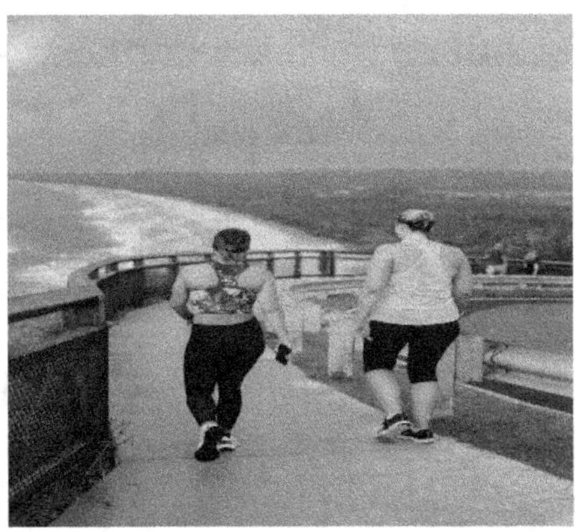

Consider when and where you may change your routine to walk instead of taking the vehicle or bus. There are many ways you can easily include this into your daily schedule.

The Benefits of Walking

- Observe an improvement in your level of fitness and muscle tone.
- Feel better and appear better
- You may notice a rise in your energy level.
- Feel significantly less stressed and become stressed more slowly.
- You notice that your sleep pattern has changed, you sleep better, and you wake up feeling more rested.
- Reduce the chance of developing heart disease.
- lessen the possibility of getting certain types of cancer

- You will discover that your depression is improving and that you are not as easily depressed as you once were.
- Your perspective on life in general and how you handle situations improve.
- You slim down and appear better.
- Your bones, joints, and muscles all seem to be stronger.
- You minimize your risk of getting diabetes.

By simply increasing the number of walks you take each day and becoming more active, you can begin to enjoy all these advantages and more.

Aim to walk at a moderate pace for the optimum benefits on your health and fitness; this implies that while you shouldn't be overexerting yourself, you should be moving more quickly than strolling.

This means that when you are moving, your temperature should rise slightly and you should be able to talk without being out of breath, but you shouldn't be perspiring heavily.

Once you've been following your new regimen for a time, you won't just feel and look better; you'll also experience a lot more health benefits and be well on your way to living a more successful, contented, and healthy lifestyle.

Benefits of Running

Running is no longer just for runners. It has been demonstrated that running simply three days a week for 30 minutes can assist maintain a healthy weight as well as boost attitude and motivation. Running, in short, can make you happier, healthier, and more successful.

- For health

Running is not just an activity for sportsmen. Whether or whether you choose to compete in races, running may be a highly beneficial exercise, even though you probably won't win the Boston Marathon. You should build up to being able to run for at least 30 minutes at a time, three or four days a week, to get the most health benefits from running.

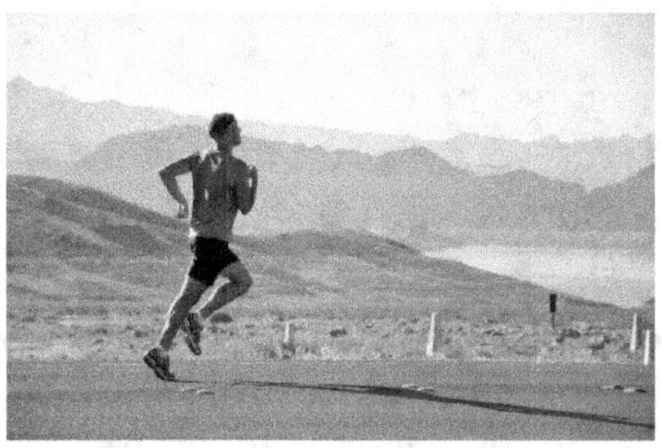

Running is the best because you can do it anyplace with just a pair of comfortable shoes. To avoid suffering an injury from the wrong shoes, visit your neighborhood running store and have them fit you. The most important thing in this situation is to have the proper footwear for your feet, not the most expensive, pricey, or nicest-looking pair of shoes.

- For Happiness

Over all other activities, running can promote a happier, healthier outlook on life. You can accomplish anything if you can get yourself out there to run three days a week. After a few weeks of running, the majority of people discover that it becomes addictive.

You will savor and long for more self-control as a result. When you get outside in bad weather and endure a drizzly or windy day, it may be gratifying. Running teaches you valuable lessons that will make you a happier person and show you that everything is possible if you put your mind to it.

If you run with a bad attitude, you'll discover that you won't get very far or that you'll walk for a significant portion of the distance. You'll find yourself telling yourself encouraging things, anticipating the hills, and convincing yourself to believe that jogging is your favorite pastime even though it isn't to persuade yourself to keep going.

You'll begin to believe it, which is an incredible thing that will start to happen. After some time, you won't have to force yourself to run; instead, you'll look forward to it and like it.

As you get to this point, you'll notice that your outlook on almost everything is more optimistic.

One of the finest ways to change your mindset is to run.

You'll find yourself thinking positively about all elements of your life, such as handling difficult clients at work, once you start to look forward to jogging up those hills since it will make you stronger and quicker.

Instead of losing patience, you'll start to consider what you could say to help them feel better so you can go on to the next client.

- For inspiration

You'll undoubtedly start to question if you could run farther or faster once you've completed the first 30 minutes of non-stop jogging. Almost every weekend, the majority of individuals can locate a 5k or 10k race within driving distance; this can help you determine how quickly you can run.

These competitions might be a terrific source of inspiration for you and your brand-new interest. Run the first one as quickly as you can; just get it done. Following that, you'll probably start trying to beat your previous performance, and you can find new races whenever you feel like pushing yourself.

Getting Fit by Cycling

You don't need to be an athlete, exceptionally fit, or anything of the type to benefit from cycling. Cycling has many advantages and is a pleasant method to obtain the fitness we all need.

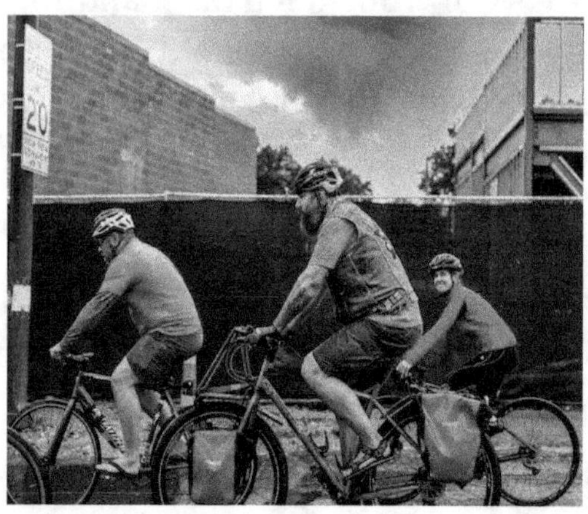

Cycling and weight loss

More exercise regularly is much more effective than diets alone for weight loss than dieting alone very rarely is.

If you bike every day, you'll not only burn a lot of calories during your workout, but you'll also increase your metabolism and burn more calories throughout the rest of the day.

Your metabolism will continue to speed along even when you stop, assisting you in burning calories more quickly. Cycling along a flat road or path at 12 mph will help you burn off about 450 calories each hour.

Cycling is good for your health and can help you lose weight and keep it off. When compared to people who don't pedal, those who bike at least 20 miles each week can help cut their chance of acquiring heart disease in half.

Health Benefits of Bicycling

Cycling is categorized as an aerobic workout; this type of exercise is very good for the heart and lungs. When you pedal, your lungs expand, allowing you to breathe in more oxygen, which in turn causes your heart to beat more quickly so that the oxygen can be distributed throughout your body.

You will be well on your road to fitness if you work on building a strong heart and lungs. Your muscles will start to tone up and you will start to feel healthier and fitter with just a few kilometers of cycling every day.

1. Cycling will have the largest positive impact on your thigh, lower back, and calf muscles because these are the muscles you utilize the most, but generally, you will feel much better.

You could discover that you no longer get dizzy when climbing stairs. The best thing is that you will like bicycling more and look forward to your next adventure the more you do it.

2. Riding a bike can help us feel better when we're depressed, stressed, anxious, or depressed. Exercise causes the release of chemicals known as endorphins into the bloodstream. Endorphins produce a happy, contented sensation and are an excellent antidote to stress and despair.

Everyone may ride a bicycle in practically any place; whether you live in a city or the country, there is always a place to ride. When you adhere to a few basic rules, it is a relatively safe sport that can be enjoyed as a family and doesn't have to be expensive.

More Simple Tips to Help You Get the Most out of Cycling

Carry a puncture repair kit at all times. A water bottle should always be carried, especially on lengthy journeys in the countryside. To make cycling simpler, keep your tires inflated to the proper pressure. Make sure you always wear a bicycle helmet out of caution. To ensure you are spotted, equip your bike with lights and reflectors at all times. Use vibrant colors or preferably reflective material when cycling at night.

Pilate Exercising for Back Pain

Becoming aware of the neutral alignment of the spine and strengthening the postural muscles that support it are the two most important things back pain sufferers can learn. A Pilates exercise routine can help persons with back pain brought on by disc and joint degeneration, bad posture, or both to relieve their symptoms.

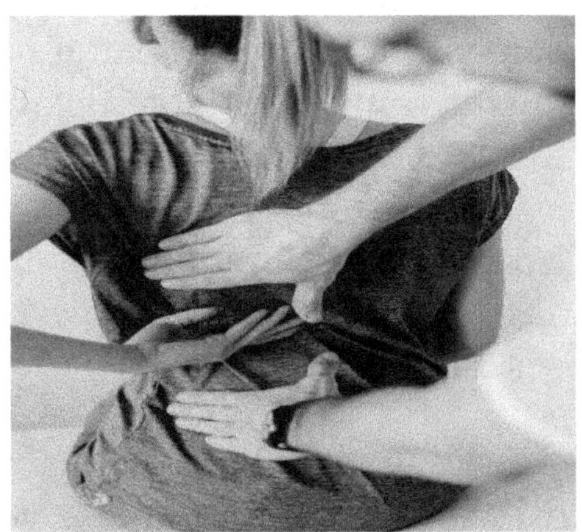

The majority of back issues are brought on by poor posture, which can occur while standing, walking, or sitting. Over time, this weakens our postural muscles, and as a result, we become unable to alter our posture even when we want to. Pilates is a fantastic form of exercise to address this issue as well.

What is Pilates All About

The Pilates technique is a type of exercise that emphasizes using the core postural muscles to support the spine and assist keep the body balanced. It is a technique that instructs in breathing awareness and spine alignment. The method not only develops the deep torso muscles but also assists in the prevention and relief of back pain.

Pilates can aid in the development of support for the deep postural muscles of the trunk, even though it is a straightforward form of exercise. It makes people more conscious of the value of neutral posture and makes the shoulders and hips more flexible.
Although some of the movements employed in Pilates, which have their origins in ballet and dance, can be very demanding and tough, other exercises can be learned and practiced at home in between supervised sessions.

The teacher leading the Pilates class should be qualified, just as it is necessary to see your doctor before beginning any new kind of exercise. One-on-one sessions might be the solution for people with severe back problems. It may be best to schedule a few one-on-one sessions with a Pilates instructor who specializes in treating back pain.

Even if it is more expensive than taking a class, getting individualized instruction might help you master the exercise correctly.

The Pilates system's exercises should push your physical and mental limits, but they shouldn't make you uncomfortable. If you are experiencing pain during an activity, you may not be completing it properly or the position may be too challenging for you.

Avoid getting physically or mentally exhausted and make sure you never put too much stress on the intervertebral discs.

In general, people who practice Pilates and have back discomfort shouldn't ever undertake any activity that forces their spine into severe extension or flexion. Spinal twisting and side-bending motions must also be avoided.

Before you see any significant changes, as with most forms of exercise, it will take persistence and some time spent attending lessons.

Chapter 5

Different Diseases & How to Combat Them

Dealing with a chronic illness will provide you with a variety of difficulties. Understanding your long-term health condition and learning what you can do to manage it can be quite helpful if you have been diagnosed with it.

How to Manage Chronic Illness

Asthma, diabetes, and arthritis are all considered chronic illnesses that may be managed with medication and medical supervision, proving that having a chronic illness does not necessarily make it dangerous or fatal.

People with these illnesses can lead regular lives and are generally healthy for the bulk of their lives as long as they take care of themselves and receive the right treatments. Even if the underlying problem is permanent and present at all times, it can be properly managed.

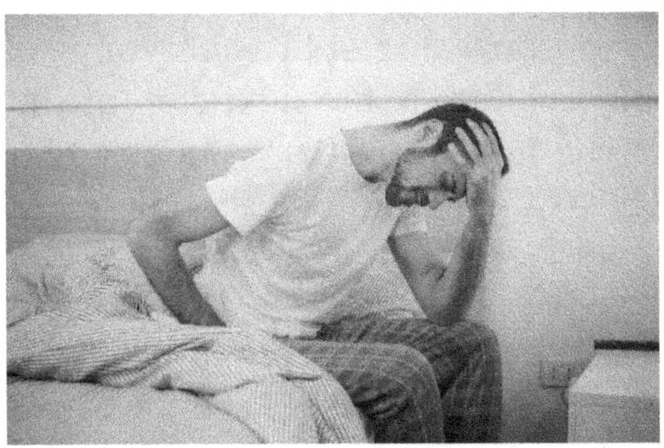

Since they feel quite well most of the time and view their sickness as more of a condition, many people who have conditions like asthma don't conceive of themselves as having a chronic condition.

However, some people experience physical, emotional, social, and in some cases financial effects. The degree to which it affects you depends on how serious your ailment is and how much therapy is required for it.

Regardless of how your condition affects you, accepting and adjusting to your chronic illness will take some time.

Whatever their ailment, everyone will go through a particular process called the coping process. Anger, worry, perplexity, and vulnerability are some of the most frequent emotions a person may experience when receiving a chronic illness diagnosis.

The need to know and study everything they can about their sickness is the next step of the coping process. By acquiring an understanding and knowledge of their condition, people can feel less fearful about it and more in control.

The third step involves gaining faith in the care they are receiving for their disease. understanding that their medication or treatment will assist in easing symptoms and episodes like those related to asthma and low blood sugar.

As the person gains self-confidence and grows more adept at managing their condition, worry and dread gradually disappear.

Everyone will progress through the phases of coping at their rate, so it's vital to recognize the diverse emotions and thoughts you have as you move through each step because they're all necessary for dealing with. You should keep in mind this advice to assist you in coping.

Accept all thoughts and emotions. It's crucial to just let your feelings come and go throughout the coping stage because you may experience a wide range of emotions. Talking with someone might be a terrific way to express your emotions.

Pose inquiries and take responsibility for your care. The unknown might be terrifying, but what we know helps us deal with it much better. Be careful to learn as much as you can about your illness.

Find out what you can do to improve your condition and what to do when it's terrible. Discuss your condition. After receiving the diagnosis, keep in mind that other family members or loved ones are likely experiencing sensations similar to yours. Don't keep your family and loved ones in the dark about your situation; talk to them about it.

Remain objective Keep things in perspective and continue living your life as you did before when you were initially diagnosed because it can be tempting to let your illness rule your life and become the most important thing.

Understanding and Preventing Asthma

An irritant typically starts an asthma episode, and irritants might differ from person to person. Asthma damages the tiny tubes that carry air into and out of the lungs.

During an attack, the muscles around the airways narrow even more, the lining swells, and sticky mucus may accumulate inside the airways, further causing more narrowing and the symptoms of asthma, mainly breathing difficulties.

Few Factors That Can Trigger Asthma

- If asthma or allergies run in your family
- Environmental elements such as variations in temperature
- Asthma in your unborn child is more likely if you smoke while pregnant.
- Asthma is more likely to develop if you smoke.
- Environmental damage
- Allergy to animals
- Asthma can start to manifest after a viral infection.
- Irritants discovered in the office

Symptoms and Signs of Asthma

The most prevalent symptoms of asthma can vary in severity from person to person; some people only occasionally experience certain symptoms while others experience them frequently. These symptoms include:

- Uncontrollable cough
- Developing a wheeze as a result of airway obstruction
- A breathing difficulty
- A sense of chest constriction

Can Asthma Be Cured?

Many different types of medications can help you successfully manage your asthma. While asthma cannot be cured, it can be successfully managed and kept under control. Depending on the intensity of your asthma, you may need to utilize a mix of medications from different categories. Categories consist of

- Asthma preventer inhalers
- Inhalers for asthma relief
- Pills of steroids
- Spacers
- Nebulizers
- Supplementary treatments

As the name implies, a preventer will help you avoid asthma episodes, so it's crucial to take it as directed every day, even when you feel OK. They often contain a very tiny dose of steroids and don't help to ease the symptoms of an asthma attack, such as shortness of breath or tightness in the chest.

Every person with asthma has received a prescription for a reliever, which works fast to reduce asthma symptoms while an attack is occurring.

If an inhaler has been recommended to you, make sure to have it close at all times.
The drug in the reliever will assist to open the airways again, making breathing much easier.

Your doctor may prescribe you a brief course of steroid medication coupled with a course of antibiotics while you battle the infection if you have asthma and are sick. Very few people who have asthma periodically need to use steroids over the long term.

Spacers and nebulizers are two methods for making it easier to take your reliever medication. Spacers are typically given to children with asthma, and nebulizers allow you to continuously inhale medication through a mask, which is useful when you are having a really bad asthma attack.

Chapter 6

Living and Managing Diabetes

Diabetes is a chronic condition that raises the possibility of developing other health issues. However, there are numerous techniques to help you manage your diabetes and continue a largely normal life.

Maintaining a healthy lifestyle, going to checkups, and effectively controlling your blood sugar levels all contribute to your ability to deal with this condition.

Checking Blood Sugar Levels

You must be able to monitor your blood sugar levels if you want to successfully manage your diabetes. You can purchase a range of household appliances that provide you with precise level indications.

The benefits of self-monitoring include letting you know when your blood sugar is too low, allowing you to check your sugar during times of illness, and giving you confidence in your ability to successfully manage your diabetes. Monitoring your levels at many points throughout the day or week is the most effective strategy to get reliable measurements.

The compact devices made for home usage are very simple to operate and come with everything you need to monitor and manage the disease.

Get Examined

Attending routine check-ups is also essential since they help prevent diabetes complications and ensure that you are successfully managing your diabetes between check-ups.
Check-ups are often performed every three months, six months, or a year.

Blood tests are performed as part of a check-up to measure your cholesterol, glucose, blood pressure, and the health of your feet and nerves. To check for any damage to the back of your eyes, you should also arrange an eye exam.

Other Dangers

You must take care of your entire health because you run a higher risk of contracting additional diseases like heart disease and circulation issues in addition to your diabetes.

Maintaining a healthy diet will greatly assist you in keeping your condition under control; you should eat regularly and include foods that are low in fat and high in fiber.

It's crucial to keep an eye on how much sugar you consume, as well as how much salt you put in your food and use in cooking.
Creating an exercise regimen is beneficial for your condition because it will not only help to maintain a healthy weight but also aid to keep your blood sugar level consistent.

You shouldn't smoke or drink alcohol if you have diabetes because doing so raises your risk of getting many other diseases. If you do drink, keep it to a minimum and avoid doing so when you're hungry because it can cause hypoglycemia.

Additionally, you should get at-home test kits for your blood pressure and cholesterol levels; if you have diabetes, your cholesterol level should be below 4.0 and your blood pressure should be under 130/80.

Carpal Tunnel Syndrome

Carpal Tunnel Syndrome (CTS) is a condition that occurs when the median nerve, which runs from your forearm to your hand through a narrow passageway in your wrist called the carpal tunnel, becomes compressed or squeezed. This compression can cause pain, numbness, tingling, and weakness in the affected hand and wrist.

CTS can be caused by a variety of factors, including repetitive motions, such as typing or using a computer mouse for extended periods, or by conditions that cause inflammation or swelling in the wrist, such as rheumatoid arthritis.

Symptoms of CTS typically include tingling or numbness in the thumb, index finger, middle finger, and part of the ring finger, as well as pain and weakness in the affected hand and wrist.
In some cases, the symptoms may also extend up the arm.

Treatment for CTS may include wrist splints, physical therapy, medications to reduce inflammation and relieve pain, or surgery to release the pressure on the median nerve.

Preventing Carpal Tunnel Syndrome

Your median nerve is protected by the bones, muscles, and other tissues in your wrist, which collectively form the carpal tunnel.

The median nerve, which supplies sensation to your fingertips, can occasionally become painfully swollen when tendons and ligaments strain against it. This results in carpal tunnel syndrome, a very painful ailment that causes your hand to hurt or possibly become numb. People with carpal tunnel syndrome frequently use their hands in the same repetitive motions.

Typists, carpenters, supermarket packers, and assembly line employees are among those who are more at risk. The syndrome is more likely to develop in those who like hobbies like canoeing, golfing, needlework, gardening, and other such activities.

It can also occur in pregnant women in the last trimesters of their pregnancies and has been connected to conditions like diabetes, arthritis, and thyroid disease.

Warning Signs You Might Have Carpal Tunnel Syndrome

- Tingling or numbness in the hands and fingers, particularly the thumb, middle finger, and index finger.
- Ache in your wrist, forearm, or palm of your hand
- At night, the numbness or agony is more intense than it is during the day.
- The more you use your hands, the worse the discomfort becomes.

- You have a hard time holding onto items and dropping them more frequently.
- Your thumb feels very frail.

To evaluate whether you have carpal tunnel syndrome, your doctor may examine your hand, fingers, and wrist.
The examination may also include a nerve conduction test.

If carpal tunnel syndrome is identified, treatment usually entails wearing a splint, resting your wrist, and altering how you use your wrist. The splint can aid in reducing pain, especially at night. Stretching activities as well as massaging the painful area and applying cold to it can all be beneficial.

There are some **things you may do to help prevent carpal tunnel syndrome**, but the problem will improve with therapy.

You may modify things by becoming more conscious of how you use your hands and tools throughout the day.

Your forearms should be parallel to the floor or slightly lowered if you stand up to work and have your workbench at waist height. Your work should be centered straight in front of you. Ensure that your wrists and hands are parallel to your forearms.

- It can help to title it if you spend a lot of time on the keyboard.
- when using a mouse and trackball, make sure to perform proper hand and wrist motions.
- make careful to maintain a close-to-sides elbow position.
- Never lay your hand or wrist on the heel, especially if they are flexed at an angle.
- A little rest should be taken every 20 minutes.
- every 20 minutes, perform some flexing or stretching exercises.

Dealing with Arthritis

Even though arthritis is typically thought of as a condition that only affects the elderly, it can afflict anyone at any age. There are believed to be more than 200 different varieties of the illness, which can affect any portion of the body. However, rheumatoid, juvenile, and osteoarthritis are the three most prevalent kinds of arthritis.

People with arthritis may experience a wide range of emotions, including rage, frustration, worry about the future, and worry about reliance.

While the illness can be crippling and makes it difficult to look on the bright side, people do adjust to the situation. For the younger person affected by the disease, thoughts like how other people will see you are a major concern.

How to Manage Arthritis

- Express your emotions and concerns

To cope with your disease, it's critical to express your sentiments openly. Speaking might help you to relieve your feelings of stress and anxiety about your situation and how other people perceive you. Your confidant can be your doctor, a close friend or relative, or even another person who has arthritis.

- Discover ways to relax and reduce stress:

Many arthritis patients find it difficult to unwind and get easily anxious. You should locate activities or hobbies you can engage in to help you relax quickly and easily or acquire routines that allow you to do both.

- Seek professional help:

If you don't feel like you can talk to a family member or friend, get professional assistance. This could be a counselor, medical professional, social worker, or resident's opinion.

The ongoing agony that arthritis causes its sufferers is one of its most crippling effects. However, patients do appear to be able to manage their pain to a point that it doesn't significantly interfere with their daily lives.

Strategies to Help Cope with and Control Pains Caused by Arthritis

To receive the most benefit from your medication, make a note of the ideal time to take it.

- Keep an eye out for when heat, cold, and resting help most.
- Examine the best workout for you and the best times to undertake it.
- Continue to use relaxing techniques.
- Take a course in pain management.
- Purchase a pain-management tool, such as a TENS unit.
- Think about getting acupuncture or hypnotherapy therapy
- Attend the pain clinics your doctor suggested.

These are just a few techniques that people have used to successfully manage their arthritis, but you should always talk to your doctor about other options.

Your doctor can also suggest clinics in your region that you can visit to learn more effective ways to manage the illness and the pain it causes.

67

Chapter 7

Alzheimer's Disease

Alzheimer's disease is a neurological condition that affects brain function and progresses irreversibly. It causes cognitive decline, memory loss, and alterations in behavior and personality. With up to 80% of cases, it is the most frequent cause of dementia in older persons. The buildup of tau and beta-amyloid proteins in the brain is what causes Alzheimer's disease.

Tau produces tangles inside the nerve cells, whereas beta-amyloid forms plaques between them. These aberrant protein buildups prevent brain cells from working normally, which causes them to die and gradually lose cognitive ability.

Alzheimer's disease normally starts with modest memory loss and confusion, but as the condition worsens, a person may have trouble speaking, making decisions, and solving problems.

Additionally, they might encounter changes in personality and conduct, as well as confusion.

Individuals may become reliant on others for their care as the condition progresses.

Alzheimer's disease currently has no known cure, therefore therapies concentrate on symptom management and delaying the illness's progression.

While counseling and support groups can assist people and their families deal with the emotional and psychological challenges of the condition, medications can also help to improve memory and cognition.

For people with Alzheimer's disease and the people who care for them, a high quality of life is essential. Early detection and treatments are essential.

Causes of Alzheimer's Disease

Alzheimer's disease is brought on by a variety of variables, and each person affected by the disease is unique. There is no one specific cause for the condition. However, advancing age and heredity are the two main variables that raise your risk of acquiring Alzheimer's.

Although this and many other theories have not yet been confirmed, it is believed that your level of mental fitness and environment may also have some role.

Who is at Risk of Alzheimer's?

By the time you are 65 years old, around 5 out of every 100 people have the condition; by the time you are 80, the likelihood has increased to 1 in 5, and by the time you are 90, over half of all adults have dementia.

Alzheimer's disease affects persons of all ages; those considerably younger than 65 have also been affected. The condition is thought to affect women more frequently than men, however, the main cause of this is that women typically live longer than men.

Genetics and Alzheimer's

Roughly 3% of all cases of Alzheimer's have a hereditary component, according to research. About 40% of those who develop the condition before the age of 65 had family relatives affected by the disease, suggesting that heredity may play a role in early disease onset.

This does not imply that having an Alzheimer's-affected family member makes you more likely to develop the disease. Contrarily, there are still steps that may be taken to assist prevent the beginning of Alzheimer's, even though people who have affected family members are slightly more at risk than others.

Preventing Alzheimer's Disease

Many people think that whether or not you are more likely to develop Alzheimer's depends on the environment in which you live. There is now research being done to determine whether exposure to specific metals plays a role in the disease's development.

Many medical professionals believe that aluminum may be the disease's likely cause and advise against using antiperspirant deodorants because of their high aluminum content.

Many medical professionals also concur that the disease's start is significantly influenced by one's mental condition. One is less likely to contract the illness the more mentally alert they keep themselves.

However, there is currently no proof that maintaining mental fitness will make a difference in either direction. Although there are numerous other potential causes of Alzheimer's disease, more research is necessary because the available data are often contradictory.

Head trauma, different viral infections, a family history of Down syndrome, smoking, and thyroid problems are among the factors to take into account.

Future of Alzheimer's Disease

There is presently no reliable test that can help doctors predict who will be at a higher risk of contracting the disease.

Researchers are focusing on Alzheimer's disease's mechanisms in the hopes of one day being able to identify those who are predisposed to developing the condition.

Researchers hope this will pave the way for treatments that can stave off Alzheimer's disease.

Managing Allergies associated with Alzheimer's

Almost everything can trigger an allergic reaction; this includes odors, foods, medications, and even animal dander.

The symptoms of an allergy can range from mild irritation to anaphylactic shock in extreme cases. Among the several groups into which allergies fall, we find:

Allergies that manifest on the skin include eczema, urticaria, and other skin rashes like hives and nettle rash.

In the summer, those who suffer from hay fever may have symptoms like a stuffy nose, itchy eyes, a cough, and a runny nose. Allergic reactions to venom include reactions to those from stinging insects and snakes.

There are a wide variety of foods that can trigger an adverse reaction in some persons. Drug allergies occur when the body has an adverse reaction to one or more of a medication's components.

A life-threatening, rapid-onset allergic reaction that affects the entire body is called ***anaphylaxis***.

Asthma is an allergy that causes breathing problems.

The symptoms of eye allergies can range from a barely noticeable itch to full-blown conjunctivitis.

Analysis & Diagnosing Allergies

If your doctor suspects you have an allergy, he or she will want to determine the specific allergen that is triggering your symptoms. A skin prick test is the standard method of identifying the allergen that is causing the reaction. The skin prick test takes only a few minutes to complete, causes no discomfort, and provides instant feedback.

The allergen is injected under the skin at a very low dose through a small needle prick; the forearm is the most common testing site. If the region where the needle was put becomes red, painful, and itching, you are likely allergic to the allergen.

It is also common for a welt to appear there. After around 20 minutes, if you still haven't had an allergic reaction, it's safe to say you aren't allergic to that particular allergen.

Dermatitis, a type of eczema, is sometimes diagnosed with a skin patch test, which involves placing patches containing several allergens below aluminum discs.

The discs are left in place for 48 hours before a dermatologist checks for adverse reactions.

Severe Allergy Cases

In extreme cases of allergy, a hospital-based challenge test may be necessary. Allergic reactions are measured when the suspicious allergens are inhaled or sneezed into the body.

A double-blind, randomized placebo test may be performed if it is thought that you may be allergic to one or more meals. Under medical supervision, you take a capsule containing the food or foods suspected of triggering an allergic reaction, and then you wait to see if you experience any adverse reactions.

Despite being the most trustworthy method, this test is only performed under the direst of circumstances due to its lengthy execution time.

Chapter 8

Dealing with Acne Problems

cne is one of those four-letter words that evoke images of unattractive skin and all the other negative connotations associated with it: zits, pimples, whiteheads, blackheads, blemishes, clogged pores, and so on. Even while it may seem hopeless, there is reason to hold out for a better future.

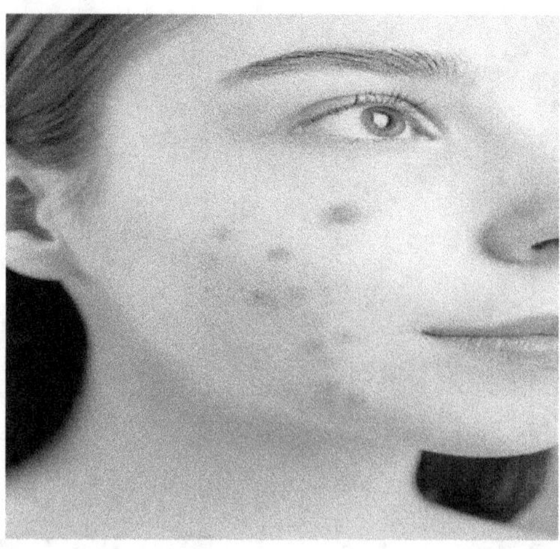

The most common acne triggers can be effectively treated. Body chemistry changes, for instance, during puberty, menstruation, and menopause, might trigger acne breakouts. Over scrubbing the face to get rid of acne and an excess of germs in the pores are two more common causes.

Natural cures, prescription medications, and over-the-counter acne treatments are all treatment options.

Common Quick-fixes At Home

Wash your face gently twice a day using an exfoliating cleanser and some anti-acne soap purchased from your neighborhood pharmacy or grocery shop. Washing first thing in the morning and last thing at night will give you the cleanest skin and hair possible. In addition, avoid picking at acne.

To cure and disinfect your skin, try a honey face mask or an anti-acne mask from the drug store. The mask can be used as often as twice a week.

Talk to your doctor about starting a daily multivitamin and chromium supplement. Keep your hair behind the ears and away from your forehead.

Take lots of water
the standard recommendation is eight glasses of water each day. And eat beta-carotene and vitamin

A-rich foods like carrots to aid with skin regeneration.

Makeup, watercolors, and the like should be applied to the face sparingly unless they are water-soluble or specifically labeled as non-comedogenic. Also, change your pillowcase frequently.

Wear at least an SPF 15 sunscreen if you must go outside in the sun. Pick one that doesn't clog pores by making sure it's not comedogenic or acnegenic. Put on a cap and some shades. avoid tanning beds as well.

Let's First Clear up Some Acne Misconceptions

Acne is exacerbated by greasy foods, stress, and chocolate. This idea is completely false. These components have no logical or scientific relationship to one another.

Zits can be reduced in size by squeezing them. It's false here as well. Squeezing can make matters worse by driving infection deeper into the skin and perhaps resulting in scars.

Acne can be helped by time spent in the sun. Not the case. Excessive exposure to sunlight has been linked to an increase in skin dryness and irritation, as well as an increased risk of wrinkles and skin cancer in later life.

Tips to Lower Your Blood Pressure

Having your blood pressure checked at least once every two years is recommended, as high blood pressure can cause health issues like blood vessel damage if left untreated.

The dangers of high blood pressure include an increased possibility of stroke, renal failure, and heart disease. It simply takes a few minutes to get your blood pressure checked, and if there is a problem, your doctor can prescribe medication and suggest lifestyle adjustments.

Here Are Some Easy Ways to Modify Your Routine and Maintain A Healthy Blood Pressure Level.

Put out those cigarettes:
Tobacco smoke causes constriction of blood vessels and an increase in heart rate, two reasons why everyone who smokes should make every effort to quit.

Quitting smoking helps lower blood pressure and reduces the risk of heart disease and heart attack even if your heart beats quicker than normal for a short time.

Slim down

Maintaining a healthy blood pressure can be aided by losing weight and increasing physical activity. The extra strain on the heart from carrying more weight raises blood pressure, which in turn raises the risk of cardiovascular disease and stroke.

Reduce your alcohol consumption:
Drinking alcohol in moderation is also recommended because, while it can increase blood pressure in some people, in others it seems to have little to no effect.

You shouldn't drink more than one glass of wine or one can of beer each day, and if alcohol use raises your blood pressure, you should stop.

Limit your intake of sodium

Sodium has the potential to raise blood pressure in some individuals. Reduce your sodium intake if your doctor has told you that your blood pressure is too high. Avoid adding extra salt to your diet and read nutrition labels to learn how much sodium is already present.

Reduce your stress level

Living a demanding life and being easily stressed can raise blood pressure, so it's crucial to find healthy ways to deal with stress and avoid letting it accumulate.

Meditation, deep breathing exercises, yoga, and visualization are just some of the self-help strategies that may be learned to assist you deal with stress.

Medication for High Blood Pressure

If your doctor has diagnosed you with high blood pressure, they may recommend medication in addition to lifestyle adjustments, which are the most effective form of treatment.

High blood pressure can be treated with a wide variety of medications. If you have a condition that can only be managed with medicine, you may need to take that medication indefinitely to maintain healthy blood pressure.

However, the odds of avoiding a lifetime of pharmaceutical use improve the sooner you begin making changes to your lifestyle to improve your health, such as quitting smoking, increasing your physical activity, and adopting a healthier diet.

Chapter 9

Treatment with Alternative Medicines

The term "alternative medicine" describes medical procedures that are not part of mainstream practice. In the scientific field of conventional medicine, alternative treatments are occasionally novel and untested, but they have the federal government's seal of approval. Additionally, they occasionally have a religious, spiritual, or metaphysical theme or component.

Here are a few well-known complementary medical treatments.

- Acupuncture

This is the practice of stimulating certain body parts with minute needles inserted beneath the skin. The most common purposes of acupuncture are pain relief and physical healing.

- Apitherapy

This method, also referred to as Bee Therapy, treats patients with honey and honeybee venom. Raw honey, bee pollen, royal jelly, and propolis are common ingredients in health, cosmetic, and therapeutic goods. Biofeedback:

Here, we're talking about a device that provides feedback on the body. The feedback aids medical professionals in charting bodily processes to aid in treatment.

The results are used to establish and then evaluate how effectively the treatment is working. These machines are used to chart internal functions with greater accuracy than a human alone is capable of. People have utilized biofeedback to treat their emotional illnesses, digestive issues, stress, migraines, and irregular heartbeats. The device makes users aware of the possibility that their feelings and thoughts may affect how they perceive their condition and available treatments.

- Chiropractics

This kind of back care, which has been around for a while, focuses on the vertebrae's improper alignment as a cause of various types of pain, ailments, and disorders.

Many also pay attention to lifestyle, general health, and stress. Generally speaking, a chiropractor gently presses different vertebrae to correct them. In addition, many aids in the treatment of conditions like arthritis, back pain, and asthma.

• Feng Shui

This concept, which includes not only the four fundamental elements of earth, fire, water, and air but also a fifth element, metal, is supposed to bring harmony into people's life. Peace and tranquility are supposed to follow when these factors are balanced throughout clutter-free homes, workplaces, outdoor spaces, and other locations.

• Therapeutic Crystals

These minerals that have been crystallized are thought to possess therapeutic properties. As a form of protection for the afterlife, they are, for instance, kept in old grave sites. Many people in the modern world think that these crystals have therapeutic powers.

For instance, some healers use charged quartz to the lower abdomen to help the area's energy return when treating stomach pain.

• Herbal treatments

Herbs, whether they are homegrown or purchased, can be applied to particular diseases to aid in healing. A mixture of witch hazel and water in a 50/50 ratio is a common remedy for acne, as are candles and scented oils with lavender scents to relieve stress and garlic applied topically to warts to get rid of them.

There are numerous further alternative medical therapies available. To learn more, use your preferred search engine.

Advantages Chinese Medicine

Chinese medicine is a comprehensive, all-encompassing system that helps promote a happier, healthier, and less stressful way of life. It is a system that has helped people for more than 23 centuries and is used to identify, treat, and prevent a wide range of diseases and issues.

The various facets of Chinese medicine all essentially rest on the same idea, Yin and Yang. This is the law of attraction: night and day, cold and warm, inner and exterior.

The Chinese believe that by doing this, we may get rid of a lot of illnesses and disorders because it will bring back balance and harmony to the body and mind.

Similar to how blood circulates continuously via veins, qi is the vital force that permeates the entire body. Problems and disease arise when this Qi is disturbed; reestablishing the Qi's flow returns harmony and eliminates the signs of illness.

Acupuncture and herbal treatments are Chinese medicine's two primary pillars.

• Acupuncture

The Qi, which travels through locations called meridian points, runs throughout the body and is the subject of acupuncture. When it is flowing freely, we are well and content, but if the channels are obstructed, the Qi stagnates and, depending on where the Qi is blocked, this causes symptoms of different illnesses.

By stimulating specific body sites, the acupuncturist can restore the Qi's regular flow, which is how it works.

• Herbal remedies

Chinese herbal medicine can be taken on its own, but it is typically given after an acupuncture session. Over a thousand common herbs are combined to treat a wide range of issues and diseases.

Two primary categories of herbal medicines are frequently utilized. These include food herbs, which are typically consumed as part of a diet and are primarily used for maintenance and disease prevention.

A doctor of Chinese medicine typically prescribes medicinal herbs, which are made especially for the patient following their needs. The patient's medical condition, the setting, and the individual's constitution make up the formula.

Medicinal herbs are frequently used concurrently with acupuncture treatments to enhance the rebalancing benefits of acupuncture. Chinese medicine offers various advantages and is said to have healed a wide range of physical illnesses as well as affective disorders and improved mental clarity.

Some Ailments it has been Proven to Effectively Treat:

- Asthma, bronchitis, and sinusitis
- Cataracts and conjunctivitis
- Osteoarthritis, sciatica, and stroke
- Quicker healing after an injury
- Better circulation
- Relief from anxiety and stress
- the absence of pain
- Increasing immune system vigor
- Eating disorders, phobias, and addictions

With Aromatherapy, You Can Improve Your Health:
Essential oils, which are compounds in their most pure form, are used in aromatherapy, a practice that dates back to 1920.

The oils are concentrated liquids made from plants using various techniques, such as solvent extraction, distillation, or expression processing. And the finished oils are then used for healing and the treatment of various illnesses.

Rene Maurice Gattefosse is genuinely responsible for the invention of aromatherapy. When his arm caught fire while he was researching the potential healing benefits of oils, he unintentionally spilled lavender oil into it, causing the limb to heal more quickly and without a scar.

Since then, a lot of research has been done on the benefits of aromatherapy for both physical and emotional recovery.

Common Uses of Aromatherapy Oils

Aromatherapy oils are frequently used as scents for homes and workplaces to encourage soothing feelings in occupants and to assist get rid of unwelcome odors and viruses.

The scent of fried onions and other foods can be eliminated from a kitchen, for instance, by lighting candles and burning wax chips produced with aromatherapy oils.

A soft scent might make individuals feel more at home after a long day at work. Bergamot, eucalyptus, lavender, jasmine, and rose are common smells.

Lavender oil is one of the oils that can help combat germs. Others, like menthol and camphor, can strengthen your central nervous system, improve your metabolism and endocrine system, and increase your immune system so you can battle colds.

Additionally, other aromatherapy oils are applied during massage therapies. The oils are absorbed by the skin and muscles, where they stimulate thermal receptors that make the muscles feel warm and tranquil.

Still, other aromatherapy oils are used topically on the skin to aid in the eradication of microorganisms and other fungi.

Other oils are used internally, where they can boost immunological function, act as a diuretic, and help with antibacterial action.

Safety Measures

utilize the following recommendations as safety precautions when determining whether to utilize aromatherapy for your diseases and healing:

1. Pure essential aromatherapy oils can be extremely potent and dangerous for you, children, and animals. So, before using aromatherapy products, carefully read the labels and, if necessary, consult your healthcare physician.

Additionally, avoid applying pure, undiluted oils to your skin.

2. If you have epilepsy, asthma, or are pregnant, avoid using aromatherapy oils.

3. Test the components and taste a drop or two to see whether you are allergic to them.

4. Aromatherapy oils should only be used sparingly because they can have adverse effects, including eye burning.

Chapter 10

How to Naturally Treat Depression Without Drugs

On the surface, it appears that trying to treat depression without pharmaceuticals is pointless, especially in this day and age when the majority of people are accustomed to receiving treatment with prescription medications.

But many people are successfully avoiding prescription medications and locating non-drug therapeutic options. Drug-free therapy, which normally has fewer side effects and is more affordable, is increasingly being used by people who are depressed.

- Low-light blues

You must select the right kind of therapy based on the root cause of your depression. You can utilize phototherapy if your depressive disorder only appears in the winter when the days are short and the amount of daylight is scarce.

It is thought that bright light therapy, or blue light therapy, administered with the aid of a lightbox would lessen or eliminate the source of this kind of depression.

- Psychotherapy

When psychological issues like distorted thought patterns are shown to have contributed to depression, psychotherapy will be beneficial. In these situations, a strong rapport and mutual understanding between the counselor and the patient will make psychotherapy or counseling more effective. Due to the patients' faulty cognitive processes, depending on the degree of the disease, lengthy and frequent counseling sessions may be required.

It is necessary to alter thought processes, interpersonal interactions, and low self-esteem. Stress must be reduced or removed, self-hatred must be transformed into self-love, and so on. In general, the strategy the counselor uses and the relationship they have with their patients are what matter most.

- Exercise

Additionally regarded as a very effective treatment for depression, physical exercise is sometimes used in conjunction with psychotherapy. It works well to relieve excessive tension, which can lead to depression.

Even though it could be challenging to get people who are seriously depressed to exercise, persistent efforts to encourage them to engage in regular physical activities are likely to be beneficial.

Group physical activities have been shown to effectively treat depression by addressing its underlying causes, such as stressful situations and tragic breakups of personal connections.

- Diet and Food

Dietary supplements, particularly those high in Omega-3 fatty acids (especially those found naturally in oily fish), can be effective treatments for depression in some circumstances. Antidepressant properties of products containing chocolate and vitamin B-12 have been established.

It has also been discovered that some herbal remedies work. The obvious treatment for depression caused by the abuse of sedatives, sleep aids, coffee, alcohol, and other intoxicants is to teach the patient to avoid these depression triggers.

- Praying and meditating

To treat depression naturally, deep breathing techniques and meditation are becoming more and more popular. These have provided highly beneficial effects, especially when used consistently for a long time. Depression sufferers benefit from meditation's calming influence on the mind.

Spirituality and prayer may be helpful in this sense as well.

Rehabilitating sad persons is a societal and familial duty. A depressed person frequently merely wants the love and attention of their loved ones. Drug therapy alone will not be able to cure depression.

Because of this, the stigma attached to mental diseases like depression needs to be eliminated. Family members must avoid making assumptions about sad persons because this could exacerbate the issue. The best place to begin your search for a depression cure is with love and support.

How to Live a Healthy Life Through Sleeping

The majority of us don't get enough sleep and are unaware of the genuine benefits it may have on our bodies and minds. While some of us struggle with sleep disorders like insomnia, others of us simply stay up too late and have obligations that need us to rise early.

For our general health as well as for getting through the day, obtaining adequate good sleep is crucial.

Our hormones, which interact with one another and have an impact on our health, are one of the largest effects that sleep deprivation has on our bodies.

Lack of sleep causes us to crave more sugar and carbohydrates, and it also causes our blood sugar levels to fluctuate.

The adrenal glands, which govern your body's health, may have issues if you don't get enough sleep. When our adrenal glands begin to suffer, we also begin to suffer.

The hormone cortisol, which is essential for blood pressure regulation, mood regulation, and stress resistance, is one of the key issues. However, an increase in cortisol can have negative effects on our bodies and is not healthy for us.

9 Ways to Get Enough Sleep

- Avoid eating before bedtime

If at all possible, avoid eating after 7 p.m., as your body will have less time to digest food before you fall asleep. Your body will spend the entire night digesting the food you consumed rather than sleeping.

Additionally, feeling uncomfortable and tossing and turning all night long will result from going to bed with a full stomach.

- Exercise often throughout the day

If you don't exercise regularly throughout the day, you won't feel weary. Regular exercise makes you fitter and improves your ability to sleep at night.

- Dim the lights:

Just as the morning sun coming through your window gives you energy, dimming the lights at night might help your body calm down and unwind.

- Purchase a comfy mattress

If you struggle to get comfortable in bed at night, think about investing in a new mattress. If your current mattress is old and worn, this may be the cause of your constant tossing and turning.

- Use a Timetable

Establish a timetable and stick to it to create a routine and a healthy internal clock. Every day, wake up at the same time, and go to bed at the same time.

- Avoid taking naps

If at all possible, stay awake during the day and avoid taking naps; doing so throws off your internal clock and leaves you feeling less exhausted at bedtime.

- Keep your bedroom uncluttered

Don't set up a desk or computer there so that you'll be tempted to use it as an office. If you have work to do, you will almost certainly be thinking about the things you have to do or should do, which may keep you up at night.

- A hot beverage

Try relaxing with a hot beverage before turning in for the night. Of course, allow it time to work its way through your body; otherwise, you may awaken with the urge to use the restroom.

- Make chocolate with hot milk if possible; stay away from coffee and tea.

Conclusion

Congratulations for making it to this part of the book. I hope the Information here will help transform your life positively. We look forward to your positive feedback.

Regards!